OUTLIVE
EVERY
PROGNOSIS

"ALL DONE! ALL DONE!"
DAVE LANGLEY

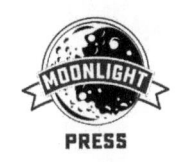

MOONLIGHT PRESS

1. Scripture quotations marked (NIV) are taken from the Holy Bible, New International Version®, NIV®. Copyright © 1973, 1978, 1984, 2011 by Biblica, Inc.™ Used by permission of Zondervan. All rights reserved worldwide. www.zondervan.com The "NIV" and "New International Version" are trademarks registered in the United States Patent and Trademark Office by Biblica, Inc.™

2. Scripture quotations marked (NIrV) are taken from the Holy Bible, New International Reader's Version®, NIrV® Copyright © 1995, 1996, 1998, 2014 by Biblica, Inc.™ Used by permission of Zondervan. All rights reserved worldwide. www.zondervan.com The "NIrV" and "New International Reader's Version" are trademarks registered in the United States Patent and Trademark Office by Biblica, Inc.™

3. Scripture quotations marked (NKJV): Scripture taken from the New King James Version®. Copyright © 1982 by Thomas Nelson. Used by permission. All rights reserved.

4. Scripture quotations marked (NLT) are taken from the Holy Bible, New Living Translation, copyright ©1996, 2004, 2015 by Tyndale House Foundation. Used by permission of Tyndale House Publishers, Carol Stream, Illinois 60188. All rights reserved.

5. Scripture quotations marked (KJV): are taken from the King James Version (Public Domain).

©2024 David W Langley
All Rights Reserved

In Loving Memory of:

Joshua David Langley

July 3, 1984 – March 23, 2016

And Dedicated to:

Anyone Who Has Ever Heard, "I have some bad news" from a Medical Professional.

Contents

Author's Foreword vii

I Have Some Bad News 1

A Father's Faith 4

Hospitals and Doctors 14

Agreeing Together 21

The Church Reaches Out 28

Night Terrors 35

The Waiting Room 39

Our Lowest Point 46

The Prayer of Faith 59

A Divine Appointment 66

Life's Journey Extended 77

All Done!. 90

Author's Afterword 95

Author's Foreword

If you or someone you love has heard the words "I have some bad news" from a medical professional, I wrote this book for you. I did not write this book to celebrate diseases, medicine, or doctors. This book is a celebration of life. A well-lived life is lived in the moment, enjoying the abundance God offers us. The question has always been how to receive as much of that abundance as possible and enjoy it for as long as possible. The world often sends things threatening to shorten our lives and destroy the joy and abundance we were meant to experience. We call those things diseases that threaten the quality and length of our lives. Diseases often reduce the time we have to enjoy the people and things we love most. With every disease a doctor diagnoses, there seems to be a prognosis. That prognosis generally speaks to how long and how well someone will be able to live with the disease if it continues. My goal is to help you reduce the impact of the disease and "outlive every prognosis."

There such a fragile balance to life and sometimes it hangs by such a thin thread. This book is about living an abundant life, which involves "outliving every prognosis" you or the ones you love have been given. What you are about to read draws on biblical truths and on a number of my own personal experiences and helped me to grow in my understanding of those truths.

What is on the pages that follow has been told and retold as a part of my oral storytelling and public speaking. My writing here is purposely conversational in style. My goal is simple direct communication of what I believe to be some powerful nuggets of truth about "outliving every prognosis." Everything you are about to read happened pretty much as it is described. In some cases, names have been changed to protect the privacy and anonymity of specific individuals.

This said, I would like to thank God the Father for being trusted to father and raise two incredible sons, Joshua and Jacob. While much of this book is about Joshua's journey, his triumphs and his shear will to live at no time do I want the message that his life preaches to overshadow the accomplishments of Jacob, his younger brother.

Jacob is passionate, hard-working, and dedicated. He is the founding member, songwriter, and lead guitarist of the pop-punk band Handguns. Through hard work and dedication, he and his band received international recognition on the alternative music scene when they were covered by

AUTHOR'S FOREWORD

Alternative Press Magazine twice in 2012. He has been involved in the music industry for nearly 20 years and has a following that covers the US and a few foreign countries. While Jake's success has made us all very proud, Josh was incredibly proud of his younger brother's fame.

I want to thank Jesus Christ, God's Son, for rescuing me from the darkness and leading me to the love of my life and the mother of my sons, Marla Kay Langley (nee Vetch). That journey to meet her took more than twenty-three years and took me fifteen hundred miles from my home near Baltimore, MD, to Bowdle, SD. I want to thank the Holy Spirit for His daily illumination of the scripture as it has applied to my life and journey and for the inspiration and strength He has provided to follow the path He has chosen for me.

I also want to express my deep appreciation to Pastor James Yutzy for his insightful comments and willingness to read the final version of this manuscript before I sent it to press.

I genuinely hope that something here helps you on your journey and that God blesses you richly as you get closer to Him and closer to home.

David W. Langley
Carlisle, PA

I Have Some Bad News

We were prepared, or so we thought. The baby's room was ready. We read all the books that new parents were told to read. Everything seemed to be in order.

The calculated day of delivery came and went. We became more anxious. First, there was false labor. Then, we were one week late. A week and a half and still nothing. The summer days were beautiful, but they seemed endless as we waited for the birth of our first child.

July 2nd came and went like any other day that summer, but by 11:58 PM, we were in the labor room. Nine hours later, we left the delivery room. We were the proud parents of a seven-pound, 13 1/2 oz baby boy that we had already decided to name Joshua. Little did we know the Jericho and the battles that little boy and we, as his parents, would face.

As they wheeled Marla from the delivery room, I went for flowers. I was tired, but I was very proud and very happy. When I returned later that morning, the flowers I carried seemed like such a small symbol of my love and appreciation for all she had been through in the preceding ten months, let alone the last nine hours. Looking through the nursery window, put a bounce in my step. By the time I reached Marla's room, I was nearly running.

She hadn't seen the baby. She had lots of questions that kept me running to and from the nursery window for answers. Hours passed, and we still had not seen or held our little boy.

Then footsteps echoed down an otherwise quiet hall. We both squirmed with excitement. As the door swung open, I jumped to my feet. It was only a nurse. I was disappointed. She had come to check Marla's vital signs. She said, "The doctor will be around to see you in just a few minutes."

That few minutes lasted TWO HOURS! When the door finally opened again, I knew something was wrong. The doctor was alone. She broke the silence with – "I have some bad news."

A pediatric emergency team was on its way. They would be taking our "baby" to a regional pediatric treatment unit in Aberdeen, South Dakota. "We just aren't equipped to handle his needs here."

When Marla asked to see him – the doctor hesitated. "I don't think that's a good idea." Her tone of voice said everything that her words didn't.

I HAVE SOME BAD NEWS

Marla broke into tears as I sank to her side in fear. "I just want to see my baby. Is that so much to ask," she sobbed as the doctor left the room.

A Father's Faith

A few minutes later, having regained my composure, I stepped into the hallway. I asked in a somewhat faltering voice, "Why won't you let her see the baby before they take him?"

"Because I don't want your wife to become too attached. It's better that way – In case SOMETHING happens." I certainly wasn't ready to consider that "something." Since that "something" in the Doctor's voice sounded ominous.

"Will it put the baby in any extra danger?" I asked, trying to restrain the anger in my voice.

"Not really."

"Then, bring him – I'll take responsibility for my wife." The "good doctor" and I had our share of prior disagreements. When Marla had an issue of blood (spotting from a urinary infection) and a false labor two weeks earlier, this woman was far more concerned about HER FEE than she was about her patient.

No one is as concerned about your health as the GREAT PHYSICIAN. I am reminded of:

A certain woman, which had an issue of blood twelve years, and had suffered many things of many physicians, and had spent all she had, and was nothing bettered, but rather grew worse, when she heard of Jesus, came in the press behind, and touched his garment. For she said, if I may touch but his clothes, I will be whole. And straightway the fountain of her blood was dried up; and she felt in her body that she was healed of that plague. And Jesus, immediately knowing in himself that virtue had gone out of him, turned about in the press, and said, who touched my clothes?" Mark 5:25-30 (KJV)

Even though the crowd that followed Christ was large, He was still personally touched by this woman's need. He felt the "virtue" that healed her go out of Him. He felt her pain as He felt virtue leaving Him, "For we have not a high priest which cannot be touched with the feeling of our infirmities" (Hebrews 5:15 KJV). While you may have been told Jesus no longer heals our diseases, "that's what He gave us doctors for," Let me assure you nothing could be further from the truth. He is "the same yesterday, today and forever." (Hebrews 13:8 KJV) He says, "For I [am] the

Lord, I change not." (Malachi 3:6 KJV) Anything God ever has done, He is still doing! The question is not whether God will heal. The question is, will we seek Him for the healing we and those we love need? This seeking means going wherever God leads us to get the help we need. It takes the type of stubborn persistence that goes to the doctor, agrees to the testing, listens to the diagnosis, considers and pursues the treatment options, presses through the crowd, and believes God for what seems impossible. Sometimes, it takes stubborn faith to get the healing we need for ourselves and those we love.

We are told that this woman sought the help of medical professionals. She had "suffered many things of many physicians." (Mark 5:26 KJV) Despite all of their treatments, some of which seemed to have been painful, these "physicians" were not able to stop her vaginal "issue of blood." No matter what the doctors did, she only grew worse. The social ostracism significantly increased the medical problems she faced since a woman was considered unclean and was expected to quarantine herself when her menstrual blood was flowing. This poor lady seems to have been menstruating for twelve years without relief. Then, the woman heard about Jesus and His Healing Power. Let me encourage you friends to get the very best medical treatment from the best doctors you can get, but if and when they run out of options, never forget "Jesus Christ [is] the same yesterday, today and forever." (Hebrews 13:8) He can heal you just like he healed a lady with an "issue of blood" that followed him down a crowded street over 2000 years ago.

> ## Like the Lady in the Crowd You Can:
> ## OUTLIVE EVERY PROGNOSIS THROUGH THE POWER OF PRAYER!

While modern medical science has made numerous advancements since Hippocrates, physicians often continue to be slow to respond to their patients on anything more than a purely scientific level. This robs them of the emotional intelligence that might result from being "touched by the feeling of our infirmities." With a great desire to diagnose and little desire to discuss their patient's concerns, these modern healers seem at times to become calloused and hardened to "the touch." While remaining detached and emotionally uninvolved is intended to keep the doctor from having their best medical judgment clouded by their feelings, it also robs them of some powerful human insight. Thank God Jesus is not calloused to our touch.

Salvation and Healing

When I accepted Christ on August 27, 1979, I received a real living Messiah who, through the power of the Holy Spirit and the prayer of his followers, still saves, delivers, and heals. Scripture does not support the modern idea that God no longer does miraculous works through his followers. Where the church no longer preaches healing in the Name of Jesus, it is generally out of fear. The fear that everyone won't be healed seems to have prevented some modern preachers from preaching the healing available for believers at the foot of the cross. Let me set your mind at ease, friend; God does not heal everyone on earth. Some He heals in heaven. And, still, others die in their sin and disease. The only reason for promoting the thought that God heals everyone here on earth is to sell a book or convince someone to spend their money on a ministry that promises healing to everyone. These promises are empty because preachers do not heal. God, however, still does. If we are willing to rely on Him, pray for the sick, and accept that He is a loving God who wants what is best for all of us, we will have the privilege of seeing (which I have had) His power work through the prayer of faith to heal the sick.

I have witnessed countless healings over my thirty years of prayer ministry. I also openly confess that I have prayed many times for people who did not receive immediate healing. The lack of noticeable immediate results does not permit us to conclude that God doesn't still heal when we offer the prayer of faith. I have believed in and preached Divine Healing since the earliest days of my ministry. I still believe in and preach it today. The only thing that has changed over the years is my understanding of how God heals, when and where God heals, and why the sick sometimes do not receive healing here on earth.

Most of us who have preached that Christ's sacrifice not only saves from sin but also heals from disease have had our faith tested. Experience says that if you preach the doctrine of Divine Healing, YOU WILL be tried. Most often, the trial comes in the form of a personal physical attack on the health of the preacher. I learned the value of both a human physician and The Great Physician (Jesus) during just such an attack while I was preaching about God's Miraculous Healing Power in Bowdle, SD, in the winter of 1982.

At the end of the evening service, I went home to my bungalow. I could tell I wasn't doing well and went to bed. The next day, I didn't go out. I stayed in bed and tried to keep warm, which was very hard given that it was winter and the bungalow had no insulation and only an oil space heater in the living room for heat.

Toward evening, Marla, my bride-to-be, not having

seen me all day, stopped by to check on me. Finding me still in my robe and not doing well, she left and returned in 15 or 20 minutes with her mother, Milda. Milda was a senior member of the congregation in which I was an associate pastor. Milda insisted that I come to stay in the spare bedroom at their house, at least until I was over the fever that I had and was in better health.

I conceded that it would be a good idea to go stay with the Vetchs. That was my last coherent decision for several days as my fever hung on and eventually spiked to 105. I have no meaningful memory of this time period. My wife and mother-in-law shared that I tossed and turned constantly and was delirious at times. They put dry sheets on the bed I slept in three times a day. I have been told by medical professionals that I have met in the years that have passed since those days that a fever of 105 in a 23-year-old male generally leads to brain damage. I certainly had my understanding and preaching of Divine Healing put to the test.

I told Marla and Milda when I agreed to stay in the spare bedroom that I did not want to see a doctor. By this point, The Enemy was already tormenting my now feverish mind with, "You said you believe that the Lord heals all your diseases." (See Psalms 103:3). This torment led me into a trap that so many believers fall into when it comes to believing God for healing. That is seeing healing as an either-or proposition. This thinking leads believers to conclude, "Either I believe in Divine Healing and I don't go to a doctor," or "I don't believe in Divine Healing and rely solely on medical professionals." This is precisely the way the enemy wants us to think. By getting us to feel like this, he convinces us to cut ourselves off from one more avenue God might use to bring us the healing we need.

I had a breakthrough in health and my understanding of healing during the winter of 1982 because my future mother-in-law insisted I see the town doctor. By that point, I was too exhausted and incoherent to argue with her. So, I took the antibiotic he gave me, and the fever broke.

Thus, through the cooperative efforts of my mother-in-law-to-be, her home remedies, the doctor, and his antibiotic, I was back in good health in a few days. Thanks to the Lord and Him alone, there was no permanent brain damage. More than anything, this experience taught me that when you seek healing for yourself or someone you love, you must be willing to explore every possible avenue because you do not know what God will use to bring the needed healing.

As you read this book, don't think that I am anti-doctor. I am not! The Bible is not anti-doctor. In fact, Jesus said, "They that are sick need a physician." (Luke 5:31). I believe that doctors serve an essential purpose in our society. They tell us what is wrong with us. Sometimes, they can fix it, and sometimes, they can't. When they can't, we can say with the Psalmist David,

> *Bless the Lord, O my soul, and forget not all of his benefits: Who forgiveth all thine iniquities and **healeth all thy diseases**… Psalm 103:2-3 (KJV)*

Unfortunately, many Christians don't seek the help of a competent physician sooner. Some seem to think that if they deny the existence of an illness, God will take it away. Nothing could be further from the truth. Much like sin, we must confess we are ill to receive healing. Please note that each time Jesus healed someone, he asked them what they wanted from Him. This was not because He did not know what they wanted or needed. It is because we are not in a position to receive from God until we confess our need. This is just as true of healing as it is of salvation. God gets no glory from us LYING about the condition of our health. He says:

> *Is any sick among you? Let him call for the elders of the church; and let them pray over him, anointing him with oil in the name of the Lord:*

and the prayer of faith shall save the sick, and the Lord shall raise him up; and if he have committed sins, they shall be forgiven him. Confess your faults one to another and pray for one another, that you may be healed. James 5:14-16 (KJV)

You must admit you are ill to receive healing, but you should not dwell on your illness. Instead, what you should dwell on is God's promise. That he is the Lord "Who forgiveth all thine iniquities; (and) Who healeth all thy diseases." (Psalms 103:3 KJV)

Hospitals and Doctors

"He is so tiny but such a beautiful baby boy. He seems so perfect. I don't understand why they are taking him." Marla said.

The emergency team nurse took him from Marla a short 20 minutes after they brought him to the room. I had been able to hold him briefly, kiss him on the forehead, and pray for about two minutes over him before I gave him to Marla. She needed to hold him. Her heart was aching. She hadn't been able to breastfeed him. She pumped milk, which they took from the room to the nursery during the day. She was aching for that connection between a mother and a newborn. I also have to believe Josh was aching for that connection.

The emergency team nurse and the EMTs with her left the room with Josh, and Marla broke out in tears. All I could do was hold her. Her sobbing was uncontrollable.

When the sobbing finally broke, the questions came. She asked, "Why my baby? Why are they taking my baby? Why is this happening to us? We're good people;

HOSPITALS AND DOCTORS

sure, we're not perfect, but what have we done to deserve this?"

I didn't have anything profound to say. It has been my experience that in cases like this, there isn't anything helpful you can say. I had learned well from one of the senior pastors under whom I interned in Baltimore before moving to South Dakota that your prayerful presence is needed more than your words or thoughts at a time like this. I was struggling enough to make sure that my presence was "prayerful." This should have been one of the happiest moments of our newlywed life – the birth of our first child – a beautiful baby boy. Instead, our joy seemed swallowed up by fear of what might come next. All I could manage at this point was to hold Marla and tell her, "We'll get through this together."

Her sobbing continued with an occasional "Why, my baby." In a while, Josh's nurse, Kathy, a long-time friend of Marla and her family, entered the room. Kathy said the Doctor is going to release you tonight. She gave Marla a prescription they had filled from the hospital pharmacy and sent her home with instructions to rest.

While Kathy was guarded at the time about what she said, later, she would share everything with us after the doctor left the community under questionable circumstances. She said that night, "There was a true knot in the umbilical cord during delivery. Typically, if they give a little oxygen to the baby in cases like this, the baby perks right up and is fine." When Kathy suggested that he should have some oxygen in the delivery room, the doctor later said no and that it wasn't necessary. When he still seemed listless and unresponsive later in the nursery, the doctor said no to the oxygen again. The doctor told Kathy, "This is what you see in babies when their parents use drugs."

Kathy got upset, "You don't know these people. I have known Marla and her mother all her life. She does not use drugs, and he is a minister." Eventually, the doctor conceded that the oxygen would do no harm. Perhaps by that point, the window of opportunity for oxygen to be helpful had passed; we'll never know. Later, we were told by both Kathy and some of the other doctors involved in Josh's treatment that we probably had grounds for a malpractice suit. While I was furious about the treatment Marla and Josh received, we did not sue this woman who professed to be a follower of Jesus Christ. We paid every penny of her fee, in time, with interest.

"Go home and get some rest, Marla. The team from St. Luke's is the best. I trust them and believe they will do everything they can for him," were Kathy's last words that night. We both understood why Marla was being released so soon. As an itinerant preacher who supported his family and ministry with the income from a small farm & home products business, I didn't have health insurance when Josh was born. This meant I had paid the doctor as much as I could in cash over the months that preceded Josh's birth. At that time, I still owed her seven hundred dollars, the rest of her fee for the delivery and well-baby care. Now, there would also be a hospital bill. It felt like it was indeed all about money. For a long time, I felt guilty about not being a better provider for my wife and our son.

We didn't get much sleep that night between the heartache, the questions, and the tears. We left home for the pediatric intensive care unit at St. Luke's Hospital in Aberdeen, SD, early the following day. St. Luke's was the largest hospital for at least a hundred miles in any direction. The trip from the small country hospital in Bowdle, just two blocks from our home, was about 55 miles. We took the same route Josh would have taken by ambulance the night before. When we arrived, he was hooked up to all kinds of tubes and wires.

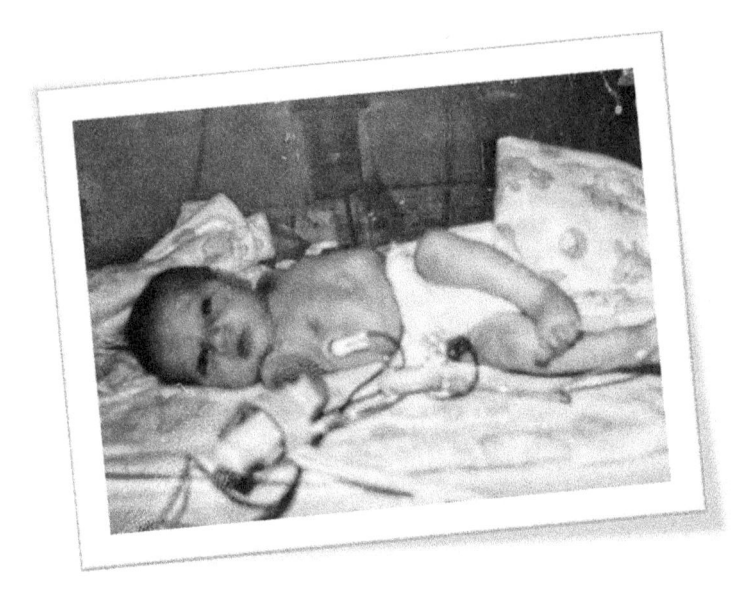

Our first picture of Joshua, complete with tubes & wires.

He seemed so little to be experiencing so much. Was he being punished for something we had done? We both had to keep fighting feelings of fear and guilt. I wondered if there was something we should have done differently that would have prevented all of this from happening to our son.

We were still not allowed to hold him. This left both of us feeling empty and aching inside. I could understand why they did not let me hold Josh, but why would they still not let Marla, his mother, hold him? All the nursing staff would say was that he had to stay in the isolette. I tried to comfort Marla, but it was almost useless. So, I stood close to her, held her close, and tried to say as little as possible. I realized she wasn't interested in anything I had to say about the situation. She was only able to feel heartache and emptiness for hours as we waited for the Doctor to meet with us for the first time.

All we could do until the doctor came was stand in our gowns with our surgical gloves on and take turns sticking a finger or two through a small window they opened in the isolette to touch his hand or arm. When it was my turn, I stroked his arm and let him grip my finger, but his grip was weak, and he seemed listless.

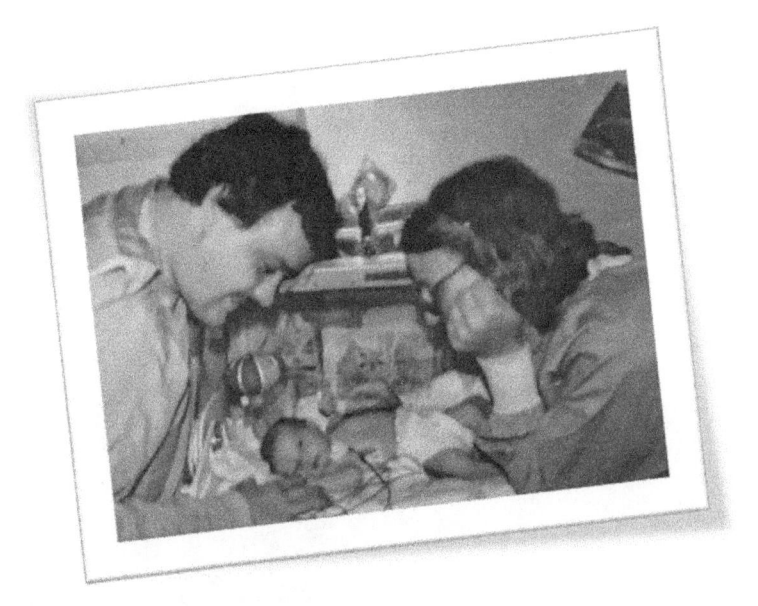

Not being able to hold Josh was the hard part for us.

OUTLIVE EVERY PROGNOSIS

Tough times come to everyone. Perhaps your tough times have not been quite like this, but before you start to feel sorry for us, please remember what happened to us can happen to anyone. We tried not to argue or be short with each other. Keeping your emotions in check at times like this can be very difficult. As we battled through the hurt and heartache, we agreed to be patient with each other, hang onto each other, and stay together until we had seen this thing through.

Agreeing Together

The hard places in life can either drive us apart or pull us together as couples. When we quit denying that our son had some serious medical challenges and we quit blaming God for not preventing those challenges, we realized that we had something special. That something special was rare among the parents we met in pediatric wards. We had a way to cope with the hardball that we had been thrown. We had the ability to agree with each other in prayer for our son. We took Jesus at his Word and began to agree with each other in prayer:

> *Again, I say unto you, that if two of you shall agree on earth as touching any thing that they shall ask, it shall be done for them of my Father which is in heaven. Matthew 18:19 (KJV)*

It was God's Love and Strength that sustained us through what were some of the darkest days of our married life. We also had the support of countless praying saints across North and South Dakota as we waited.

As new parents, we initially wanted to believe that there was nothing wrong with Josh. Faced with traumatic news reports like those we were receiving on a minute-by-minute basis during those first eight days of Josh's life, we reacted the way many people do when faced with terrible news. First, we denied that there was anything wrong with Josh. He seemed so perfect just looking at him. Maybe he was a little sluggish, but he was a newborn. When the doctor finally came in to do her rounds, we were told they would run a series of tests on him. Based on the pre-admission notes from the doctor who delivered Josh and what they had seen so far, she believed he was limp and unresponsive as a result of an "inborn metabolic error."

I could tell she was still guarded about what she said but was not encouraging. I could also tell the information that she was fed by the doctor who delivered Josh was probably clouding her judgment as well. I felt sure that the country doctor shared her theory with the city doctor that Joshua's ailments were a result of substance-abusing parents. She eventually allowed Marla and I to hold Josh and feed him through a feeding tube inserted through his nose and down into his stomach.

Eight days passed, one minute at a time. There was test after endless test. Followed by meeting after meeting with the doctor or medical staff. Marla and I were there together for all of it. I sold spices, seasonings and extracts, and household products off the back of my truck when I could, but I refused to leave Marla alone for any of the endless tests or treatment meetings. All of this was far too difficult for one person to handle alone.

Occasionally, Marla would fall asleep during the day in a rocker near Josh's isolette, and when she did, I would sneak out for a little while and try to sell. I was 50-60 miles away from my regular farm route customers. This meant calling on new customers in a new area. It was harder to sell as much as I was used to selling to my regulars, but without me on the street selling something, we had no income.

Getting a good night's sleep was difficult in the hospital. We weren't willing to leave and at the time really could not afford to stay somewhere else. The staff let one of us sleep in a recliner next to Josh's crib at night. This guaranteed Marla a safe comfortable place to sleep. I slept where I could and when I could. Usually, this meant sleeping in a waiting room and trying to make sure that it wasn't a problem. Pediatric Intensive Care Units, I soon discovered, are used to parents not wanting to leave their child, so they didn't give me any problems and eventually gave me pillows and a blanket and showed me a waiting room that was private and dark after visiting hours. The stress, the crying out to God, the praying, and the lack of sleep were starting to wear us down.

I noticed this most when having to deal with the doctor. My patience was starting to wear thin at times. She seemed to see Josh's case as hopeless. She kept saying each day during her rounds, "He is hypotonic. He has no muscle tone. He will probably always be limp and lifeless."

She said this again and again over the first two days Josh was hospitalized. When asked why she thought that she said, "The test results are inconclusive, but I believe that what your son has is an inborn metabolic error. I believe that is why he is limp, lifeless, has no sucking reflex, and is unresponsive to normal stimuli." I had disagreed with the doctor on a number of things, but I had managed up to this point to hold my tongue. On the third day. I had finally had enough of her discouragement.

"I'm certainly not a medical professional, but I am also not an idiot either, doctor. You've been pumping phenobarbital into a seven-pound baby through an IV for three days now and you're shocked that he seems limp and lifeless? Hook that IV up to me for three days and even at 250 pounds, I'm going to be tired and out of it. What are you expecting here Doc?"

"Well, one of the nurses witnessed what she thought was a seizure when they brought him in the first night," was her response.

I said, "Only ONE NURSE saw what she thought might have been ONLY ONE seizure. Hmm! I bet if you take him off of that phenobarbital, he will perk right up."

"He needs to be weaned off," she said. The fact that he had to be "weaned off" makes it clear that phenobarbital is a powerful barbiturate that is narcotic. While it is used to treat seizure disorders like epilepsy, there was no real evidence Josh needed this powerful drug. Over the next five days, she backed off on the phenobarbital, and just as I suspected, our son started to show more signs of life. Part of praying for someone you love is also being willing to stand up for them when they can't stand up for themselves. I'm not quite sure what might have happened had I not spoken up. I only know that he started to come around more and more as she weaned him off the phenobarbital.

Just when we thought the waiting would never end, the doctor told us we could take our son home. She couldn't tell us what was wrong with Josh, but she admitted that he had started showing signs of life. She cautioned us not to "expect too much" and told us he would probably "remain floppy and would probably never walk or crawl."

When I asked if she would circumcise him before we took him home, she wanted to argue with me about how she didn't feel like that additional trauma was necessary at this point. When I pressed her, she eventually conceded, and

OUTLIVE EVERY PROGNOSIS

a female Jewish doctor circumcised Joshua on the eighth day. This didn't seem significant at the time. Still, about two years later, when Marla gave birth to our younger son, Jacob, in a birth center run by two Jewish midwives, they offered the name of a doctor and that of a *mohel*, either of whom could perform the circumcision. We chose to have the *mohel*, a Jewish minister trained in the practice of circumcision, to perform Jacob's circumcision. This Jewish Holy Man invited us into his home on the eighth day of Jacob's young life, where, at our request, he did a full *brit milah* "covenant of circumcision" ceremony.

After seven days of testing, the doctor still could not tell us what was wrong with Josh, but her pet theory was still that this resulted from an "inborn metabolic error." She kept saying, "I just can't prove it; everything we sent to the Children's Hospital in Kansas City lab came back inconclusive. I believe the test results are inconclusive because testing for this type of disease is so new that the testing tools have not been perfected enough yet." So, while there was no actual proof, only the doctor's opinion Josh's discharge diagnosis was "inborn metabolic error." This was the diagnosis that got his medical bills paid.

The nursing and social work staff were very helpful during this season of our lives. St. Luke's Hospital's Public Relations Department asked if they could photograph us for an advertising piece they were doing on the new $1,000,000 isolette that had been Josh's bed for the first eight days of his life. Joshua was literally the first baby ever to use it. Below are the pictures they took.

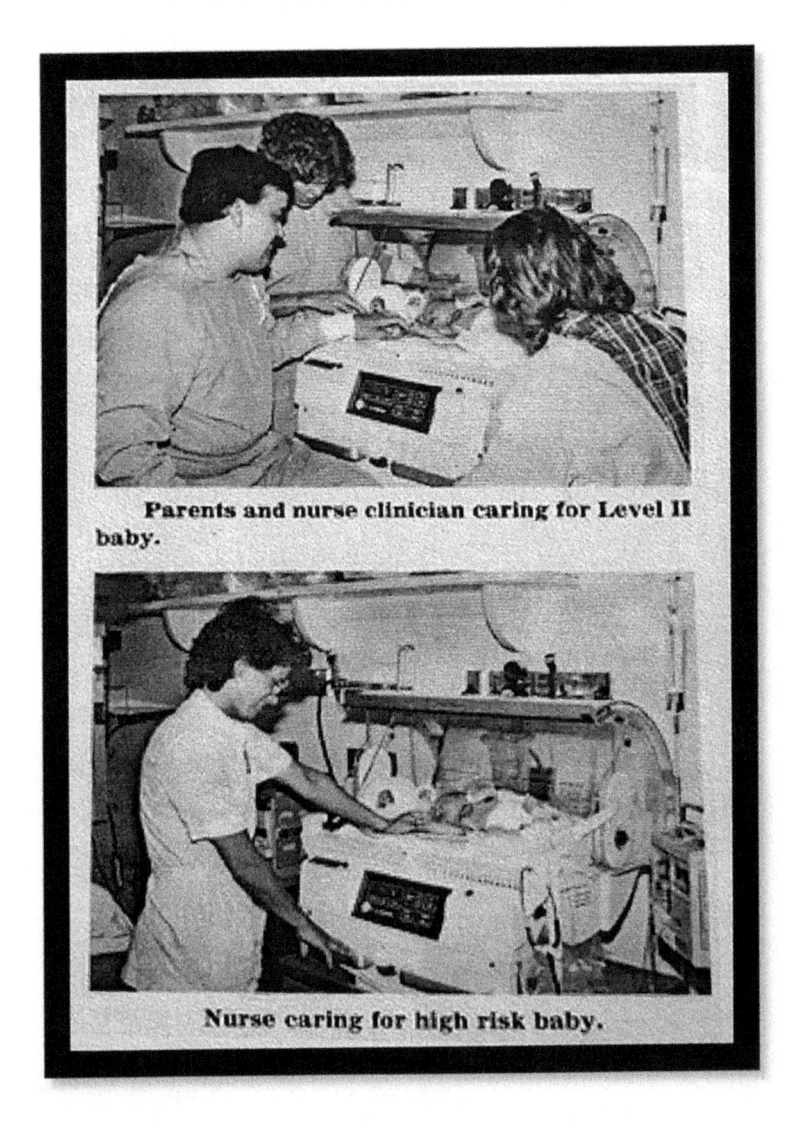

Parents and nurse clinician caring for Level II baby.

Nurse caring for high risk baby.

The Church Reaches Out

We were so thankful to be going home, even though we knew there would still be challenges. Josh was going home with an infant heart monitor, strict instructions about feeding him, and a long list of other instructions. This was by no means a normal homecoming for baby and mama. It was at least a homecoming, though.

It almost seemed foreign when we returned to our apartment above the old grocery store on Main Street in Bowdle. While it was only eight days, each one of those days seemed endless, and overall, it felt like forever since we had been home. We tried to settle back in. I put up a sign I had been working on before Josh's birth for the farm and home products business. I organized my office and tried to get back into a routine. I had a pile of paperwork to deal with, sales calls to make, and business and personal bills that needed to be paid. Marla set to work settling Josh into the nursery. We were both tired but happy to be home.

We were also so thankful to be back in our home church and surrounded by people we knew and loved.

These were people we knew had been praying for all three of us. This church family and Marla's extended family would be a strength to us countless times and in numerous ways over the next few months. We could feel God's presence in the expressions of love from that little church family. The church was to us what the church is supposed to be. When and where the church is what the church is supposed to be, the church grows. And that little church started to grow.

What the Church Should Be

Jesus told His followers what the Church should be on two separate occasions and in two separate passages. As a bi-vocational minister, I have spent my life taking my business to the marketplace and the message of Christ to the world. My years in marketing and small business have taught me that what Jesus gave His disciples on those two occasions when taken together, is what our modern marketing firms would call a positioning statement. A positioning statement is written to help define "the position" a business or an organization wants to occupy in the public mind. Below are the two "pigeonholes" Jesus said the church should occupy in the public mind.

First and foremost, Jesus said Christians should be known by their love for each other:

> *By this shall all men know that ye are my disciples, if ye have love one to another. John 13:35 (KJV)*

In short, the Church is called to be a people of love. We are supposed to be people who love and care about each other and who reach out to each other with concern during difficult times. John was right when he wrote, "Beloved, let us love one another, for love is of God; and everyone that loveth is born of God and knoweth God." (I John 4:7). Some of those people with whom we attended church probably didn't realize they were doing just what Jesus said. While they were reaching out and loving us, God was showing up on the scene and loving us, too. Where God's people show genuine Love, He shows up and shows off His life-changing power. Where people need healing and salvation, or God's intervention in a crisis situation, if we show up and show our love, our God will still "show up and show off" His Miracle Working power.

Secondly, and certainly just as significant to the future of the church, Jesus said the church should be known as a house of prayer:

> *¹² And Jesus went into the temple of God, and cast out all them that sold and bought in the temple, and overthrew the tables of the money-changers, and the seats of them that sold doves,*
>
> *¹³ And said unto them, It is written, My house shall be called the house of prayer; but ye have made it a den of thieves. Matthew 21:12-13 (KJV)*

In short, the church should be a place where the world can find people who love each other and pray for each other. This is the kind of warm, loving environment where miracles can happen and lives can be changed. If you have been blessed to experience or be a part of a body of believers like this, then you know what a powerful difference it can make in a life.

During some of those meetings in our home with believers from our church and at church services and social gatherings, we had a lot of seasons of prayer for Josh and a lot of opportunities to praise God for Josh's progress and improving health. When those friends praised God and rejoiced with us, something else miraculous started to take place. God showed up in our home and in the life of our son in so many small and big ways. Why did God show up? It certainly wasn't that there was anything special about us, our home, our friends, or the prayer that we offered. God showed up because, as the psalmist David speaking to God says,

> *But thou [art] holy, [O thou] that inhabitest the praises of Israel. Psalms 22:3 (KJV)*

Did you catch that? If you want God on the scene, start to praise Him. He'll show up when we truly praise (thank) Him because he "inhabits" our lives through the praise (the thankfulness) of his people.

If that praise or prayer takes place with other believers, He offers the following promise of His Presence.

> *"For where two or three are gathered in my name, there am I in the midst of them." Matthew 18:20 (KJV)*

The answer to all of our needs is found in His presence. We don't need to learn how to pray more eloquent prayers. What we need to do is praise Him. Invite His Presence through praise and wait on the move of the Holy Spirit. As we offer up our praise, God's presence will touch earth's praise. And, when that happens for that special moment, His Kingdom has come, and His Good and Perfect Will shall be done.

So now you're thinking, what about those times when you just don't know what to say or how to pray? Believe me, I understand. When circumstances are difficult, you may not know what to say or how to pray for someone you love. Don't let this stop you from showing up and providing the support of your "prayerful presence." There are times when a loving listener with a hug is enough. Then there are other times the Holy Spirit may intercede through us with groans and an unknown heavenly language for which there are no human words. Paul speaks of this when he says:

> *Likewise the Spirit also helpeth our infirmities: for we know not what we should pray for as we ought: but the Spirit itself maketh intercession for us with groanings which cannot be uttered.*
> *Romans 8:26 (KJV)*

OUTLIVE EVERY PROGNOSIS

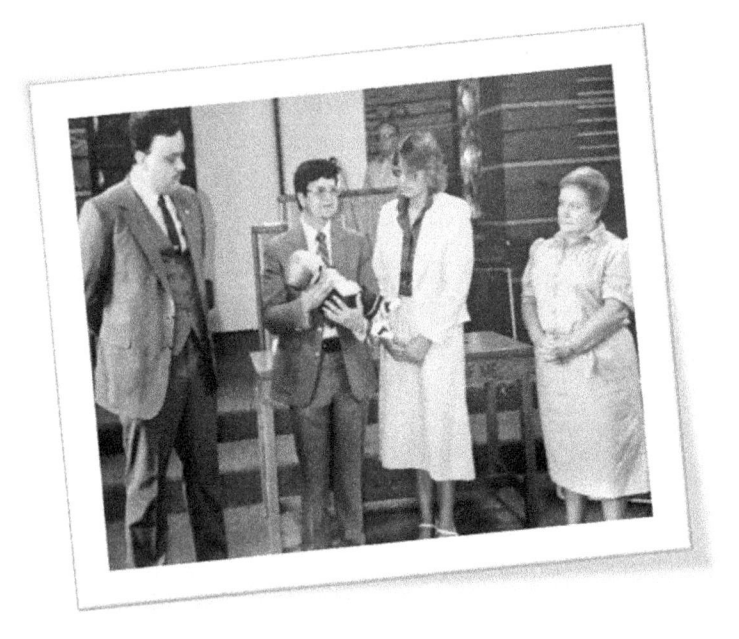

Pastor Sam Saylor helped us Dedicate Josh to the Lord as my mother, Wanda Langley, and the congregation watched!

Night Terrors

The enemy of our soul, Lucifer, Satan, or The Devil, is not only REAL but also a sly old fox that likes to terrorize God's sheep by night. While you are told, "greater is he (The Holy Spirit) that is in you than he that is in the world" (1 John 4:4 KJV). Make no mistake, Satan (the fallen Angel Lucifer) is quite powerful, much more powerful than any human operating in their human flesh. Christ defeated Satan on the cross. Satan was cast down from heaven to the earth. When he was thrown down, he took a third of the angels in heaven with him. This means that he has only limited power and limited forces. These limitations lead him and his demons to use fear as their number one tactic of warfare. In a very real sense, The Devil is the Original Terrorist. We will talk more about this terrorist, his tactics, and spiritual warfare in a later chapter. For right now, it is enough that you know he and his demonic forces strike when we are most vulnerable, and his number one tool is fear. Nothing can strike fear into the heart of a parent quicker than the prospect of the sudden death of a child.

When we brought Josh home from the hospital, we were told that he would need to sleep at night attached to an infant heart monitor. The prospect of having your child be so much at risk for crib death that one of these monitors would be necessary would strike fear in most hearts. They taught us infant CPR and sent us home with a monitor. The shrill, startling sound that the monitor produced when it went off, which it often did at night during those first few months, helped me understand what those who suffer from night terrors must go through. If Josh stirred too much, he sometimes pulled one of the electrodes loose, and the alarm would go off. When it went off, we went running. Before long, we were so conditioned to that sound that, at times, we ran before we were even awake! Once or twice, I remember being so startled that I stood straight up in our bed before taking off for the nursery.

Then, there was the colic that caused Josh to cry without stopping until his stomach pains were soothed. In large part a result of his being tube fed, because he still had no sucking reflex, the colic hung on for months and months. Between false monitor alarms and the colic, we got very little sleep for those first six months Josh was home from the hospital. Limited sleep and being startled late at night can create its own brand of fear and terror.

The only thing that seemed to comfort Josh when he was colicky was to bounce him while walking with him. This was far too hard on Marla's back; she had been thrown from a horse as a young girl and suffered almost constant back pain, so I drew most of this duty. His stomach pains were worst at night, during the time I would have liked to sleep, but I was just happy to have our little guy home and making progress. So, tired or not, I would walk and bounce Josh while offering simple sentence prayers. Paul said we should "pray without ceasing" (1 Thessalonians 5:17 KJV). I believe he is talking about maintaining an ongoing conversation with God. This involves inviting God into the moment-by-moment of your daily muddle and mess. This ongoing conversation can provide clarity to your mind, strength, help, and direction to your life every step of the way. I thank God for being there, talking with me, working in Josh's body, and helping me as I walked the floors with Josh many a late night.

We took Josh back for his first visit with the Doctor in Aberdeen about two weeks after his release. During her examination, she leaned over him while he was lying on the table. He must have seen her shiny gold necklace because he reached up and grabbed it and almost ripped it off her neck. I have to confess. I wasn't very nice. I said, "Wow, how about that muscle tone, Doc," she just shot me a glare and said, "Well, it's more than I would have expected."

The truth of the matter is she hadn't expected much. As we found out later from a county health nurse who was on the staff at the hospital during Josh's first eight days, the doctor didn't expect him to live. "And, neither did we." This nurse told Marla, "The doctor thought you and your husband would take the death better at home." What the nurse said next even cleared up why the doctor didn't want to circumcise Josh before his discharge and why nothing was encouraging in her discharge prognosis. "The doctor didn't think he would live more than a month" were her last words to Marla.

What the doctor may or may not have told the nursing staff was that she thought I was a religious nut. I thanked the doctor for all she had done when she released him to go home with us. I told her that I sincerely appreciated her help and believed she had given him the best medical attention available. I remember that she wasn't too pleased when I said, "As a doctor, you are good at diagnosing and telling us what is wrong with us. Sometimes you can fix it, and sometimes you can't. When you can't, I know someone who can."

The Waiting Room

Most of us don't like waiting. It seems like life drags on when we have to wait. Between waiting for hours in waiting rooms with Josh to see the doctor for 15 minutes and waiting on the Lord to step in and do what no man could, we did a lot of waiting in those days. The scripture promises us, though, that: "They that wait upon the Lord shall renew their strength ... "(Isaiah 40:31 KJV) The Lord knew we needed a renewal of our strength.

For the first three months, Josh was home; he was fed breast milk through a tiny tube that we inserted through his nose into his little stomach. This was because, at birth, he had no "sucking reflex." This meant Marla had to pump breast milk, which was poured into a large plastic syringe attached to the feeding tube. This made feedings a lot of work. They wanted us to feed him every two hours since he was under the desired weight for his length and age. Some days, Marla felt like all she did was feed, clean up, and get ready to feed again. This was tiring for her, and the tube feeding was causing the colic that kept me up walking the floors with him at night. We prayed and asked God for help, but the doctors offered little help or suggestions.

God can and still does at times heal someone in a moment; over thirty-two times in the New Testament, *Iaomai* or *Iama* are translated as heal to describe this type of sudden and miraculous healing. There are many times, though, when the healing He brings us comes through the path of wisdom imparted to the sufferer or someone called to minister to the sufferer. This type of healing is more therapeutic and comes over a more extended period. Yes, God uses various types of therapy to heal the sick. One of the three words translated in the New Testament as healing is the Greek word *therapeuo* from which we get our word therapy.

We had been praying for months that Josh would begin to drink from a bottle but had seen very little progress in this area. After over two months, he still had no sucking reflex. During a season of prayer, Marla began to think about how she fed "bottle calves" on the family farm when the mother cow refused to do so or couldn't produce enough milk. Sometimes, these little calves were not aggressive enough to work their way into the mama cow, or in other cases, the cow could not produce enough to feed all her calves. Either way, the calf would have starved without being bottle-fed.

By working with Josh like she had worked "bottle calves" on the farm, Marla eventually got Josh to drink from a bottle. This is an example of the gradual healing that sometimes occurs when we allow God to direct us. God always prepares us for what He directs us to do. As a farmer's daughter, Marla was prepared by her work with little calves to offer some creative in-home therapy to our son. God always provides wisdom when we ask for it and always prepares us for the work He has set us apart to do.

> *For we are his workmanship, created in Christ Jesus unto good works, which God hath before ordained that we should walk in them. Ephesians 2:10 (KJV)*

Gaining weight was a slow go for Josh, and the doctors were constantly concerned about his failure to put on weight during those early months; we continued to thank God for what we had. Our son was home with us; he was drinking from a bottle, and he was becoming livelier and showing more muscle tone with each new day. Every time we shared our praise reports with believers, they rejoiced with us. Those same praise reports shared with Josh's country and city doctors were generally met with retorts like, "Well, I wouldn't get your hopes up too much."

A Bump in the Road

We hit a bump in the road when Josh was about nine months old that might have caused us to wonder if the doctors were right had it not been for our faith and willingness to hold onto the promises of God. While Josh was drinking milk from the bottle regularly, he started to sound very congested. We thought, at first, it might be just a cold. When we took him to his doctor in the country, she said we needed to take him to Aberdeen. She thought that it sounded like pneumonia in his lungs. Her suspicions were verified by chest x-rays at St. Luke's, followed by his admission into the pediatric ward. After two weeks at St Luke's Hospital in Aberdeen, during which time Josh's health continued to decline, his pediatric specialist could not determine why he was not responding to treatment. She really seemed to be reaching her limit with what she could do for Josh. She wanted to send us on with him to the University of Minnesota in Minneapolis. She gave us his chest x-rays and told us that we should report to the pediatric neurology unit.

> *Medical Doctors serve an essential purpose in the world. They diagnose and determine what is wrong with us. Sometimes they can fix it, and sometimes they can't! When they can't, I know someone WHO STILL CAN - Jesus Christ of Nazareth!*

Waiting on the Lord

Whether meeting with her at the hospital or going to her office, which we had been doing regularly for the last nine months, this pediatric specialist could be particularly depressing. Sitting in a sea of discouraged parents all waiting to take their child into a small room where the doctor would generally offer them the worst-case scenario cast a cloud of hopelessness over the folks we met while we waited. Those other parents we met while waiting seldom knew anything about God's ability and willingness to heal the sick in response to prayer. Many of these new parents had no spiritual resources upon which to draw. During Josh's second hospitalization in Aberdeen, I discovered that the parents we met were pretty open about sharing their child's medical challenges with someone else who they sensed had a child with similar challenges. When they shared their child's needs, we always offered to pray with them. I don't ever recall anyone refusing prayer. I'll admit that a few were a little surprised when we prayed quietly but prayed aloud in a waiting room. This raised a few staff eyebrows on more than one occasion, but I was beyond the looks and the doctors who shook their heads. At Aberdeen, during that second hospitalization, we were able to pray with a new mom for her son, who was in the ward with Josh. The pediatric specialist for our son and hers walked in on us in a hospital waiting room while praying with that mom. There was no one else in the room at the time. I felt someone walk into the room before I saw her. I continued praying quietly but still aloud. The doctor paused, I finished praying, and she cleared her throat and shook her head. She had some news for the other mom, and we excused ourselves. Eventually, that mother, whose son shared a room with Josh, committed her life to Christ. That young mom not only accepted Christ but also, for several years, she and her family went on to attend church in Aberdeen with one of Marla's sisters.

In more than 35 years of Spirit-led prayer/ministry, I can't remember more than a handful of people who refused to let me pray with them when I asked, "Is there anything I can pray with you about?" In the early days, I was sometimes uncertain how people would react. Over time, having experienced their responses and witnessed some of the miraculous results God delivered, I quit worrying about what someone might think and cast all hesitation aside.

People are looking for answers to their needs and problems, and most are unwilling to rule out any avenue that might meet their needs. I will also admit that some onlookers have made snide remarks, cursed at me, and called me various names. The message here is simple: love people and be willing to pray with and for them. When you yield to the leading to ask someone if there is anything you can pray with them about, you open the door to a God moment for them and you. In those God moments, He often shows up and shows off by meeting their need.

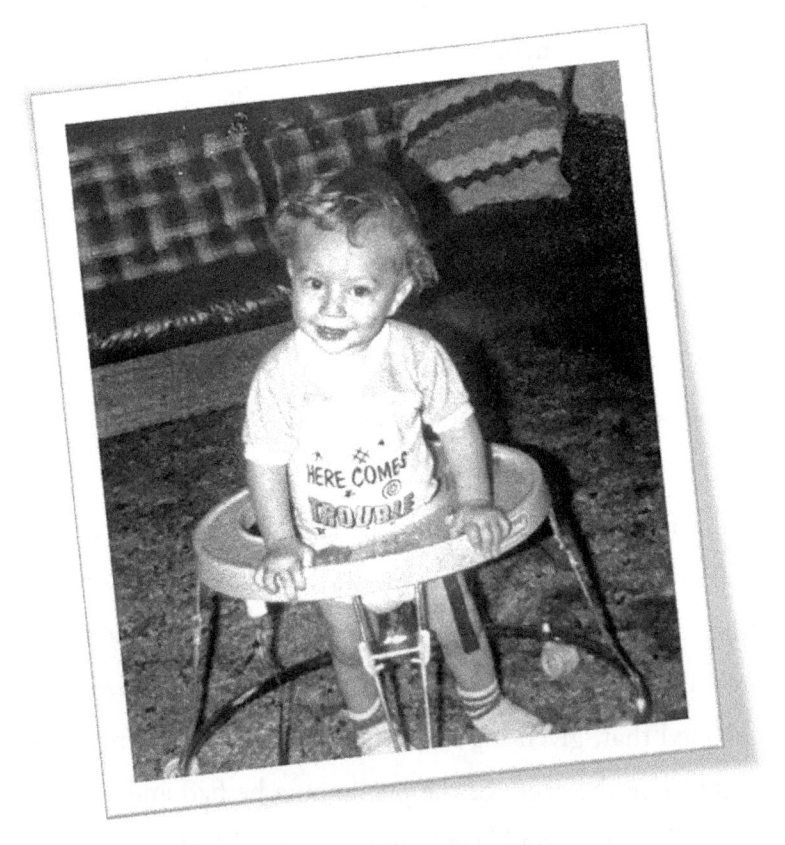

Josh at between 9-12 months

Our Lowest Point

We went back to Bowdle, packed some things, took care of some details, prayed with our church family, and, within three days, were on the road to Minneapolis. As instructed, we reported to the University of Minnesota Pediatric Neurology Department with Joshua and his chest x-rays. For a while, this had the doctors in Minneapolis scratching their heads. His paperwork said that he was suspected to have an "inborn metabolic error," which needed further diagnosis. Therefore, he was assigned to neurology, but he had pneumonia and chest X-rays.

After I explained Josh's history, they made a call to Aberdeen. When we talked with them later the first day, they seemed more up to speed on the pneumonia and the request for further testing for a metabolic error. They explained that, given his present health, they would need to determine the cause of the pneumonia he had and treat it first. Then they could begin doing some of the tests his specialist wanted them to do to determine why he was hypotonic, had low muscle tone, and had no suck reflex at birth.

As we prayed and our church family prayed with us, the doctors began diagnosing. Regarding the pneumonia, they determined that Josh was getting the milk he was drinking from the bottle into his lungs. Using liquid barium and what in 1985 was a very sophisticated piece of x-ray video equipment, they could show us what was happening when Josh swallowed. What we could not have known or seen before that moment was that, although he was taking milk from the bottle just fine, the tiny muscle at the top of his windpipe, called the epiglottis, was not closing up properly and capping off the top of the windpipe. This was allowing milk to enter Josh's lungs. That milk was continuing and would continue to create chemical pneumonia every time he was fed. The simple explanation was that while Josh's muscle tone had improved dramatically over the last eight months, the epiglottis was still too weak to protect his lungs.

We asked, "What therapy, medication, or surgery is available for a weak epiglottis?"

They said, "THERE IS NO THERAPY, NO MEDICATION, and NO SURGERY for a weak epiglottis."

I asked in a somewhat faltering voice, "So what then can you do for our son?"

The head resident in pediatrics said, "The only solution is to have Dr. Legend (not his real name, but his work in neo-natal surgery is truly legendary) insert a Gastrostomy Feeding Tube through the wall of your son's stomach!"

We both shrunk, leaned into, and held onto each other at the table. We were crushed by the doctor's words. After a long pause, I looked around the table and asked the entire team, "Are there no other options?"

I got a unanimous, even if it was a bit apologetic, "No."

"How long would he have to be fed through that tube?"

"INDEFINITELY!"

Marla sobbed, "Will he ever be able to have anything by mouth?"

"NO, it wouldn't be safe. As he grows, you will be able to feed him formulas and pureed foods through the tube. You may use sponge swabs to swab the inside of his mouth so that he doesn't lose his taste buds. Perhaps someday there will be a cure for this, but we have nothing else to offer now."

We both left that meeting in tears. Marla and I started to use a pay phone. I dug in my pockets for change, and Dr. Mac, the unit's head resident, said, "Come with me, folks." He took us to a quiet room where doctors dictated their notes at the end of their rounds. There was a phone there. "He handed us the receiver and said take as long as you want, folks." After he left the room, we both broke down into tears. Eventually, we called Marla's mom and explained what we had just been told. We prayed over the phone, and she promised to tell everyone we knew so they knew how to continue praying for Josh and us.

Have You Been Sleeping in the Hospital?

We had only had enough money to make the trip to Minneapolis and back and little for food. That meant there was nothing for a hotel room. There was no Ronald McDonald House in those days. What we did find, though, was some compassionate and caring doctors like Dr. Mac. I was thankful we did not have to pay to use the phone. Long-distance calls over landlines in those days were expensive. Dr. Mac met me in the hallway when we came out of the room after that call. He asked, "Have you been sleeping here in the hospital?"

"Yes, is that a problem?" I said respectfully but with some concern. One morning before this conversation, I had unintentionally scared a cleaning lady when she found me asleep behind the closed door of a hospital waiting room down the hall from the Pediatric Neurology Unit.

"No," he said. "But, come with me." He led us back through a hallway and showed us where the doctor's shower rooms were for the ward. "If you want to shower or clean up while you're here, just tell one of my nurses, and they will let you in and get you towels or anything else you need." I choked back tears and thanked him for his concern for us. Just writing about this thirty-nine years later touches my heart. When you reach out to families in crisis, sometimes even your smallest acts of love and kindness have long-lasting effects. His concern for our well-being in this act of kindness made it very touching. Years later, I remember a ministry friend who liked giving gift cards to restaurants and convenience stores that sold gasoline to people who had to spend lots of time in hospitals with family members. What a tangible way to let people know you care when you don't know how to extend your arms beyond your "prayerful presence."

We had previously been told that the hospital would allow one parent to sleep in a rocker beside the child's bed in the ward. They also had two mattresses they would put down as pallets on the waiting room floor for the first two lucky parents who signed up after 4 PM daily. With more than 25 patients in the ward, there wasn't much room for being late to sign up. Once I missed it because we were in a meeting. So, I snuck into another waiting room down the hall after visiting hours had ended at 8 PM. I turned out the lights and closed the door behind me. I was so exhausted that I fell asleep in two stuffed chairs I pushed together. On this occasion, an upset cleaning lady woke me up at about 5 in the morning.

The next time I missed the sign-up was a couple of days later. We were at Josh's barium swallow. After the episode with the cleaning lady, I was concerned about causing problems with the hospital, so I locked the doors and slept in the truck on the bridge that crosses from the University Hospital over to Hennepin Avenue, the heart of Minneapolis's drug and prostitution district. I'll admit that it's not a very safe place to sleep, even in 1985. The area reminded me a little of some of the Baltimore streets I had left not so many years ago. I remember that night, thinking about how far I had come in the last six years. A little over six years before that night, I was running the streets of Baltimore, in and out of the same kind of strip clubs, bars, and live sex shows that Hennepin Avenue had to offer.

Up until August 27, 1979, I lived life for myself and not for Christ or His Kingdom. I was an alcoholic with almost a fifth of bourbon per day habit. God miraculously delivered me from drinking. By the Power of the Holy Spirit living inside of me and overflowing me daily, I had been able to live in victory over alcohol, tobacco, and porn for six years. With all we had been through, it might have been easy that night to give in, pitch everything, and return to the life I once knew. It was waiting right there, just across the bridge. What kept me that cold night was love for my wife and son, love for The Lord and all He had done for me, and the realization that I had come too far to turn back now!

> *Brethren, I count not myself to have apprehended: but this one thing I do, forgetting those things which are behind, and reaching forth unto those things which are before, I press toward the mark for the prize of the high calling of God in Christ Jesus. Ephesians 3:13-14 (KJV)*

While I knew the road ahead might not be easy, the road behind me went somewhere I no longer wanted to be. I began thanking God for all the ways He had abundantly blessed me. I thanked Him for my beautiful wife, who was sleeping safely in a rocker beside our precious son upstairs in the hospital, not too far behind me. Six years ago, I couldn't have got a nice girl like her to go out with me, let alone marry me. While prayerfully concerned about Josh's health and future, I knew God was bigger than anything we faced. I had firsthand knowledge of a God who delivers, heals, and saves people daily. I knew He had brought me this far, and I felt sure He wanted to use Josh's life for His Glory. I just wasn't sure how or what that would mean.

"Aw done! Aw done! Aw done!"

The pediatric specialist in Aberdeen had Josh assigned to neurology because she believed that Josh had more significant neurological or metabolic issues. She wanted them to test for things she could not because she did not have the equipment, tools, or staff to test. Since he was the charge of Pediatric Neurology, they delivered the news to us about the barium swallow and continued testing for metabolic and neurological issues. For days while we were waiting for Dr. Legend and the gastrostomy surgery, the neurology team seemed to be constantly poking him with needles for blood for this or that test. Waking him up to take a temperature, check his vital signs, or give him this or that shot. That's not to mention the EKGs, EEGs, and hooking him up to all kinds of equipment. The nurses knew this was all uncomfortable for him, so when they were finished, they often said, "All done."

Despite his developmental delays and minimal efforts at speech up to this point, our nine-month-old, who had taken all this like a trooper, started mimicking the nurses and saying, "AW DONE, AW DONE, AW DONE!" anytime a nurse came near his bed. He wanted them to know he was already done. Josh had a fantastic sense of humor, and even in the crib, he kept us, the doctors, and the nursing staff laughing. The laughter seemed to lighten the mood a little, but nothing made the heartache go away.

As we entered the second week of Josh's hospitalization, we were becoming more and more exhausted. It was at this point that my mother flew from Baltimore to Minneapolis. She got a hotel room near the hospital. She sent us to the hotel while she spent overnights in the rocker beside Josh's bed. This was good because it meant we could finally get a good night's sleep. It had been weeks since we had one of those. Two weeks in Aberdeen and now a week in Minneapolis. I'm not sure how many hours we slept that first night, but I am pretty sure neither of us moved.

Eventually, the Neurology Staff called us in for a meeting. They had been unable to determine the causes behind Josh's low muscle tone and other neurological symptoms. They did determine that there was not anything to support the idea that this was a metabolic error. So, they settled in on a clinical diagnosis of cerebral palsy. Dr. Mac said he wasn't comfortable with CP as a diagnosis. In a real moment of sincerity, this man I had come to appreciate so much said, "I don't think you will really ever know what the root issue is with Josh's health. I think he will be one of those kids that the right technology and testing will come along too late to give him an accurate diagnosis. In the meantime, his symptoms fit CP, so we call it CP because, without a diagnosis, insurance will not cover his treatment.

The tone in the room was both uncertain and depressing. "Without a diagnosis, I guess you just treat symptoms as they arise?" I asked.

"Yes, that's correct."

"So even though you don't have a diagnosis, what would you say is a reasonable life expectancy for our Josh?" I asked, and then I squirmed. There was a long silence, during which everyone at the table looked at each other, almost as if to say, "Are you going to answer that?"

Finally, the woman who was Head of the Pediatric Neurology Department said, "If he makes it beyond the first year, survival rates increase dramatically, but still, I would be surprised if your son lives beyond his teens. I doubt that he will make it to 21."

Meeting a Legend

I remember the first time we met Dr. Legend (not his real name). He was followed by an entourage walking two or three steps behind him. As one of the premier pediatric neurosurgeons in the world, he was more than a doctor. He was indeed a legend. As we would soon learn, other

Doctors, often including department chairs, had to bow to his decisions.

Dr. Legend said he had reviewed our son's file and, "We will be inserting a tube like this one through the wall of your son's stomach." He had one of his residents hold up what looked like a foot-long length of quarter-inch rubber surgical tube. This will allow you to feed him milk, formula, and pureed foods in time. He asked if we had any questions. It was hard enough to think about our son not eating like healthy children ate; we couldn't come up with any questions.

"We will come for him early tomorrow morning. It won't take long. I'll come out and see you after I'm done," he said, and just as fast as he came, he and his entourage left. The whole meeting might have lasted 7 or 8 minutes.

As promised, they arrived the following morning to pick up Josh and take him to surgery. We went to the waiting room outside of the Pediatric Neurosurgery Suite. About 45 minutes after they wheeled Josh into surgery, Dr. Legend came out and told us, "The surgery was uneventful." The tube was in the wall of his stomach. He told us the staff on Josh's ward would teach us how to manage feeding him. Dr. Legend shook our hands and said he wanted to see Josh in three months.

The Tube

Josh's lungs were clear; he had a new diagnosis and a new piece of hardware to manage. We referred to it as "the tube." This was to go along with the infant heart monitor, or just "the monitor," as we called it, that was waiting for him back at home. The treatment team in the Pediatric Neurology Unit taught us how to manage his feeding tube and prepared us for Josh's discharge. While we were glad to be going home, it was also a little hard to say goodbye to the staff, who were starting to feel like extended family.

The trip from Minneapolis to Bowdle was long. So, we stopped around 2 or 3 in the afternoon in Milbank, SD. We asked for a booth in the back corner of the restaurant; we were both hungry, and Josh needed to be fed. We ordered our meal, which came quickly, so Marla ate quickly, and then she laid Josh down on the booth seat beside her. Her back was to the back wall of the restaurant. There might have been 5 or 6 other patrons in the 30' x 40' dining room. We were both struggling with being forced to feed Josh this way. It was awkward and embarrassing, so Marla tried hard to be as private as possible about what she was doing. I purposely moved to block the view of anyone behind us sitting at the counter.

I hadn't finished my meal when the restaurant manager came to our table and said, "Folks, I'm going to have to ask you to leave. We have had some complaints that what you are doing is disturbing some of our patrons." Okay, I said, we'll go. Marla was almost done feeding Josh. She stopped, taped the tube to his side, and packed up. Then, we headed for the door. Marla went to the truck to finish Josh's feeding.

When I got to the counter with the check in my hand and money in my pocket that my mother had given us to get home on, I said to the manager who was standing at the cash register loud enough for everyone in the restaurant to hear, "We're leaving, but I just want you to know you people have bigger problems than my son. And, oh by the way," looking at the manager, "I'm not paying for this meal." This was the first but certainly not the last time I had to stand up for our son in a public setting. People can be so brutal about what they don't understand.

When I got to the truck, Marla asked me, "Were you respectful?" As a child at home, she was taught to avoid strife at all costs. I started the truck. I said, "Yes, but it was hard. I wanted to do and say a lot more, but I limited myself to telling them that 'they had bigger problems than our son and that I wasn't paying for the meal' since they asked us to leave. In a few more hours, we were home.

The Prayer of Faith

Returning home meant adjusting to a day-to-day routine, which, while it would be a comfort, would also be a challenge. In addition to the infant heart monitor, we would have to come to terms with "the tube." The thought of tube feeding was scary and embarrassing. We loved our son; I loved my wife, and I didn't want to see either of them deal with potential ridicule over something that people like those we met in Milbank wouldn't understand.

We continued to pray and to try to believe God for a miracle for Josh. I frequently found myself praying and saying to the Lord, like another father we meet in Mark Chapter 9, who brought his son to Jesus. That father said,

> *"Teacher, I brought my son, who is possessed by a spirit that has robbed him of speech. Whenever it seizes him, it throws him to the ground, he foams at the mouth, gnashes his teeth and becomes rigid. I asked your disciples to drive out the spirit but they could not."*

> "You unbelieving generation," Jesus replied, "how long will I stay with you? How long shall I put up with you? Bring the boy to me."
>
> Jesus asked the boy's father, "How long has he been like this?"
>
> "From childhood" he answered. "It has often thrown him into fire or water to try to kill him. But if you can do anything take pity on us and help us."
>
> "If I can?" said Jesus, "Everything is possible for one who believes."
>
> Immediately the boy's father exclaimed, "I do believe, help me overcome my unbelief."
>
> Mark 9: 17-24 (NIV)

Reading this passage repeatedly during the days that followed our return home, I saw parallels between this story and our situation. I repeatedly confessed my belief despite all the professionals who, like the disciples in this passage, could do nothing to help. I needed the Lord to "take pity on us and help us." Based on all we had been told and all Josh had gone through, I needed his help with any remaining unbelief.

I went back out selling on my farm and home products route during the day. I had a lot of financial catching up to do. I had been gone from home and my business for over a month, but I would not change anything about having been there. I believed that God could and would help us make up our losses. We received several generous gifts from some family members, church members, and community members who had heard about our plight. Someone even paid a huge heat bill we had fallen behind on while we were away taking care of Josh. Word traveled fast in our rural area; most of my customers, even though some of them were 25 to 30 miles away, heard about our situation, and they were ready to stock up, which helped bolster our sales until we could recover some.

We were still praying together as a couple for Josh. We had some church friends and family members continuing to pray with us for something more complete in the way of healing. It was hard; I preached Divine Healing, and I believed in Divine Healing, but why wasn't my son completely healed?

This was a recurring question. I found myself reading and rereading the passage in Mark, trying to figure out why, in this tough case like ours, the disciples could not cast out the spirit and heal the child. King James says that Jesus told his disciples, "This kind come forth by nothing, but prayer and fasting." (Mark 9:29 KJV) I knew that the NIV translation team and many later scholars did not include "fasting" because, according to their scholarship, it did not appear in the earliest manuscripts. So NIV says, "This kind comes out only by prayer."

While I wrestled with this and other passages covering the issue of Divine Healing, Marla was doing some wrestling of her own. She began thinking about how, if what we were told was true, Josh would never taste a McDonald's cheeseburger. She cried out to God for understanding, and God led her to James Chapter 5 as a part of her morning devotions, while "I exclaimed I do believe; help me overcome my unbelief."

One evening, when I came in from work, Marla announced that we needed to have the elders of the church pray for Josh. I knew instantly that she was referring to James 5:14-16, where James writes:

> *Is any sick among you? let him call for the elders of the church; and let them pray over him, anointing him with oil in the name of the Lord: and the prayer of faith shall save the sick, and the Lord shall raise him up: and if he have committed sins they shall be forgiven him. Confess your faults one to another, and pray one for another that you may be healed. The effectual fervent prayer of a righteous man availeth much. James 5:14-16 (KJV)*

I knew the passage well; I had preached from this text years ago when I got sick and my fever spiked to 105. I had always believed in the prayer of faith. I had seen and participated in this practice in Maryland before I moved to South Dakota. I had to admit that while it was a part of the Pentecostal Churches I attended in the East, I had not yet seen it practiced in the Church of God in South Dakota. Doctrinally, we said we believed in it, but in most of our local churches, we seemed to have quit believing in its power.

I said, "I don't know if we could get our elders to do that, honey."

"I don't care if they want to do it or not. They're going to do it. I am sick and tired of this." Marla was insistent.

"Okay, we'll talk to them on Sunday."

We arrived at church early Sunday morning. We asked to speak with the pastor. I was not on the church staff at that time, I had helped the pastor and served as an unpaid associate in our small congregation. Marla just blurted right out what she wanted, "I want you to arrange for the elders of the church to meet here at the altar after church and to anoint Josh with oil and pray the prayer of faith over him."

I can't say I know where they got the oil to anoint Josh. I know when those three farmers came to the altar, they all seemed pretty unsure of what this was all about, what they needed to do, and what was supposed to happen. I remember the pastor and I both explaining a little bit about the prayer of faith as James described it. I don't think any of them impressed me as knowing or believing that Jesus Christ still healed the sick today. They joined us at the altar, anointed our son with oil, and began to pray. Today, I couldn't tell you who led that prayer, how long it lasted, or what was said.

I remember that three men willing to honor God in prayer for healing in the life of a young, helpless child did what they were asked to do. God honors prayer when it honors Him. God honors us with His Presence when we acknowledge the truth and authenticity of His Word. The King James Version of the Bible says that "the elders" are to pray the prayer of faith, and it "shall save the sick, and the Lord will raise him up; and if he have committed sins, they shall be forgiven him" (James 5:15 KJV). When I read James 5:15 in the New International Version after that prayer service, I realized what I had been missing all along. The New International Version (NIV) reads, "And the prayer offered in faith will make the sick person well; and the Lord will raise them up. If they have sinned they will be forgiven." The critical difference here is that we are to confess our need to the elders of our church. While it is not their responsibility to heal us, we are told that their prayer, offered with a belief in the truth of God's Word found in this passage, is all the faith it takes to touch God's heart.

James goes on to write later in the first half of verse 16 of this chapter,

> *Confess your trespasses to one another, and pray for one another, that you may be healed. James 5:16 (NKJV)*

This verse makes it clear that sometimes, even after the prayer of faith, more may be required to receive the healing we seek. It may not be enough to confess your need for healing; you may need to confess your sins. This confession should be heard by a fellow believer. James then unleashes a solemn promise on us in the second half of verse 16:

> *The effective, fervent prayer of a righteous man avails much. James 5:16 (NKJV)*

A Divine Appointment

In the days that immediately followed that prayer, it would have been easy to become discouraged because, at first, nothing seemed to be different about Josh. We continued to feed him through the tube. He continued to sleep with the heart monitor, and life seemed to be pretty much the same as before we asked for prayer.

Then something rather unexpected and frightening happened. Josh was becoming more and more active, but he was still behind in his development. As a ten-month-old, he should have been, but he was not yet crawling. Instead, he would roll from place to place. At first, this was exciting, fun to watch, and sometimes funny. Like the time he rolled down our home church's carpeted center aisle. The pastor, seeing Josh, chuckled and said we have been called "holy rollers" before. Go ahead and roll, Josh. (In the early 1900s, during the Pentecostal outpouring from which our denomination sprung, it wasn't uncommon for members of other churches to call us "holy rollers." They also attempted to stone our preachers for their preaching during camp meetings on the Baptism in and Gifts of the Holy Spirit.) Then, laughing, he said, "If someone were to walk in off the street and see Josh rolling down the aisle, they really would believe we're 'holy rollers' and that we start them young." The whole congregation laughed. It was nice to feel at home and loved by God's people. Later, Josh rolled into a clean trash can that he knocked over at Grandma and Grandpa Vetch's house. He laughed and laughed and laughed. Notice the gauze and tape on his side, which covered and held the gastrostomy tube in place.

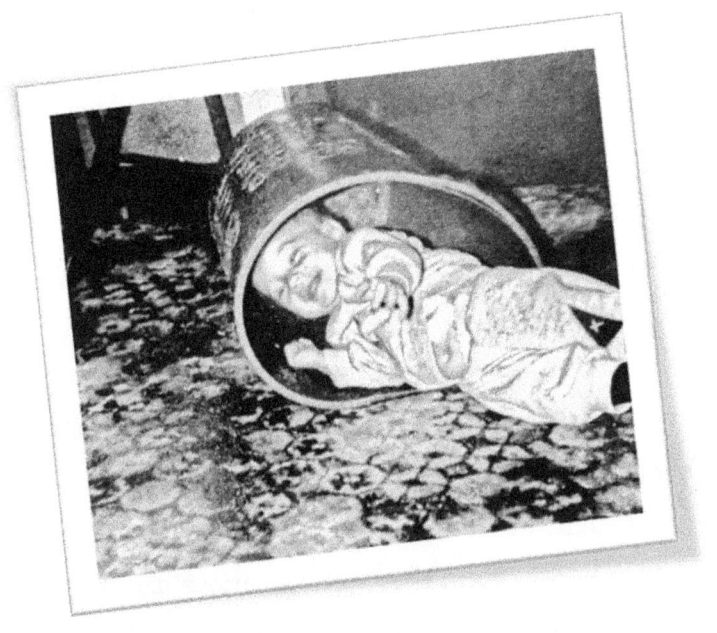

Josh is laughing and rolling inside a clean trash can that he knocked over at Grandma and Grandpa Vetch's House. Notice the white gauze and tape on his side covering the gastrostomy tube.

We were starting to have some happy memories with Josh until one night, while he was rolling on the floor in the living room, we heard a loud pop from his stomach. When we turned him over, the tube had come out of his stomach. We needed to get him to the hospital in Aberdeen, 55 miles away. We called ahead, told the ER what was happening, and left immediately. When we arrived at the ER, they took him straight into a surgical suite where a radiologist they had called in from home did as he was instructed over the phone by one of Dr. Legend's residents. He inserted a smaller tube in the incision in Josh's stomach through which we could feed him until we could get him back to Minneapolis. He told us we needed to get him to Minneapolis so that Doctor Legend could do the job properly as soon as possible.

The next morning, we called to see if we could do his twelve-month check-up sooner and explained what happened to the University of Minnesota staff. We were told we might have to wait to see Dr. Legend, but he would get to us when he had an opening.

We were thankful that nothing serious had happened when the tube popped out, according to the Doctors in Aberdeen. So, at eleven months old, Josh was on his way back to Minneapolis for another checkup. Stressful, yes, but something seemed a little different this time. A feeling of peace and calm was settling in over us.

When we arrived at the University, some three hundred miles from our home, we were taken into an examination room, where we were told we would need to wait. They told us that it would probably be quite a while before Dr. Legend could see Josh but that the head of Pediatric Neurosurgery would be in shortly to examine him.

We waited just a few minutes, and the door swung open. We were both surprised. It was Dr. Legend with one of his interns, "So is this Baby Boy Langley?"

We both, in unison, said, "Yes."

"So, how is he doing?"

We tried to explain what had happened with the rolling and the tube. Then Dr. Legend asked Marla, "Has he had anything by mouth?"

She said, "No, just the swabs," which were tiny sponges on a stick that we were told we could flavor to keep his mouth stimulated.

"Oh, I'm sorry," she said, "that's not completely true. My dad doesn't listen. I guess he's a grandfather. He has given Josh little licks of ice cream, too."

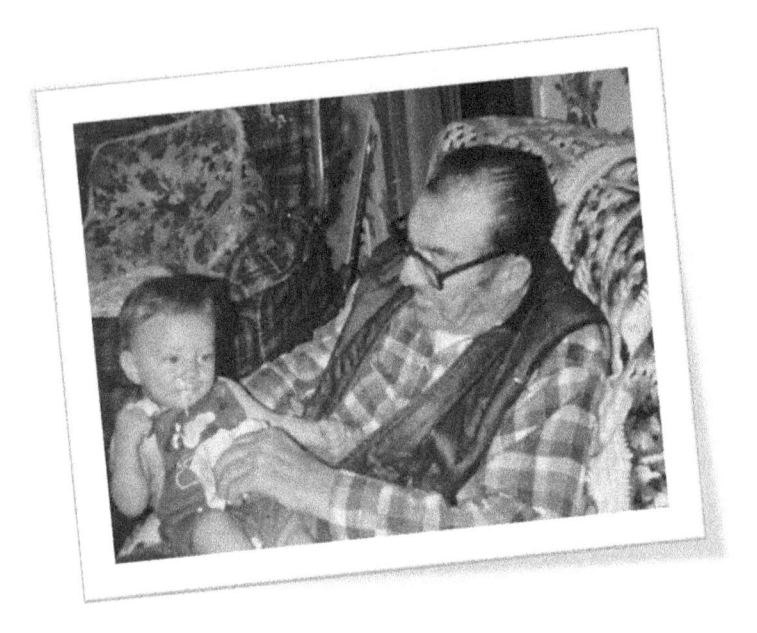

Josh and Grandpa Vetch caught sharing an ice cream neither one should've had. Grandpa had diabetes.

We weren't sure what to expect next. Dr. Legend just smiled. Josh was on the table where Dr. Legend was examining him. Then, a hush fell over the room. Everything seemed to slow down and take on a certain glow as the Dr. said, "I think your boy is going to be alright." And then, he said, "We're going to take this tube out and send you home." What happened next thirty-nine years later still blows both of our minds. I had seen God do some genuinely miraculous things in prayer lines as we prayed for the sick, but never had I seen anything more miraculous than what took place in that examining room. When the doctor reached down and pulled the tube out of Josh's stomach, it felt strangely like things I had seen happen as I assisted Dr. E.L. Terry in prayer lines during the three weeks of revival services he held in Lansdowne, MD. Not since those days as a young ministerial intern had I seen God move so conspicuously through one man as he ministered. This was indeed a Divine Appointment that I believe came in answer to the prayer of faith offered by those three men in Bowdle. There was such a Divine Visitation of God's presence that it was like watching the Hand of God reach down and touch our young son. The doctor turned to his intern and said, "Cauterize that incision," and headed for the door.

Before he could leave the room, we both thanked the Doctor profusely, and I remember saying, "Josh will be a year old next week. You have given him the best birthday present ever." With that, he was gone as quickly as he came. The resident finished and was gone for about 15 minutes before the Head of Pediatric Neurosurgery entered the room.

She launched into her brief examination. She asked a few questions but had no new thoughts about Josh's case or a more conclusive diagnosis. Eventually, as she was finishing up, she said, "It will probably be a while before Dr. Legend is able to see him."

Marla quickly said, "Dr. Legend has already seen him," and then, excitedly, said, "and he thought Josh would be fine. He said that he didn't need the tube anymore. And, he removed it."

"He did what?" In startled disbelief, the Dr. raised Josh's shirt and saw that the tube was gone.

"Did he do a new barium swallow? To verify his theory. No, of course not!" she said with frustration.

"He's not just Dr. Legend. He's GOD! Nobody dares to question Dr. Legend," she said as she shook her head. "I hope your son is really alright, but I've got to tell you I am not comfortable with this."

We took Josh home that day. We were so excited. What happened in that room that day changed our lives forever. While Josh would need speech therapy, physical therapy, occupational therapy, and learning support when he reached school age, he was able to graduate high school on time, drive his own car, and even have a brief learning-supported college experience. What happened that day in that little examining room, I genuinely believe, extended Josh's life beyond any doctor's wildest estimate. First, they said he'd be lucky to make it a week! God proved them wrong! The doctor in Aberdeen told her nurses maybe he would live a month! God proved her wrong! Finally, the best guess they could offer when the pediatric neurologist at the University of Minnesota said that he didn't believe we would ever have a proper diagnosis was that he would be fortunate, given his development and symptoms, if he made it past the first year of life to last to age twenty-one! And God proved them wrong one last time and gave him over ten more years than they thought! He proved them all wrong by "outliving every prognosis." God let us have the privilege of being Josh's parents for over 31 years before he decided Josh's work on earth was done and took him home.

> ## Like Josh You Can:
> ## OUTLIVE EVERY PROGNOSIS THROUGH THE POWER OF PRAYER!

Not only did Josh have a fantastic sense of humor, but he had a real heart for ministry. These two things made two recurring topics of conversation for Josh and me. As for that sense of humor, Josh truly liked those McDonald's burgers his mom wanted him to be able to try. I remember one occasion when Josh and Jake were still in car seats, hearing Josh say from the backseat, "Dad, let's go to McDonald's."

I said, "No, son, we don't have the money for that right now."

Without missing a breath, he turned to his brother and said, "Even the birds sing Dad's praises – Cheap, Cheap! Cheap, Cheap!"

Everybody laughed except me. I just squirmed and shook my head. Although, I must admit it was hilarious. Since that day, I have occasionally received reminders from my household that I am "just cheap!" Marla told me years ago, "You just need to let the boys have this 'cheap thing' and not argue with it. There isn't much they can tease you about, and you are cheap anyway!"

As for his heart for ministry, he would frequently ask, "Dad, when are you going to go out preaching again?"

I always responded, "When God opens the doors for me again, Josh." Right now, buddy, I'm praying for people and helping our pastor build a strong local church. During most of his growing up years, I worked as a printer and ministered around the table in our home, around the altar at Bethel Assembly of God, or preaching to drug addicts, alcoholics, and street people at Grace & Hope Mission in Baltimore's famed red-light district known as "the Block."

He remembered me preaching revivals and special services in local churches in South Dakota and briefly, after we moved to Pennsylvania. One of the speakers at Josh's memorial service, Pat King Fiske, still to this day, credits a 4-year-old Josh for bringing her to the altar at a revival I preached where she accepted Christ. Over thirty-five years after accepting Christ, Pat has lived and worked for Him as an Emmaus and Credo Team member and Leader. Josh loved seeing people get saved. As an elementary school special needs student, he rode a van to school and was brought back by van. He witnessed, frequently, to drivers and students on these buses. Twice, Josh shared his faith in Christ with two different female bus drivers on the ride home from school. Each time, he popped off the bus and said, "I told her mom, I told her." Each time, the bus driver was in tears, and Josh went off into the house to get his after-school snack while Marla was left to pray with the driver.

After graduating from high school, he briefly attended a learning-supported college program at the Hiram G. Andrews Center in Johnstown, PA. It was during that season of his life that he began to struggle with what seemed to be years of anxiety and emotional turmoil. Life had not ever been easy for Josh. He was a brave fighter and fought for life on a daily basis.

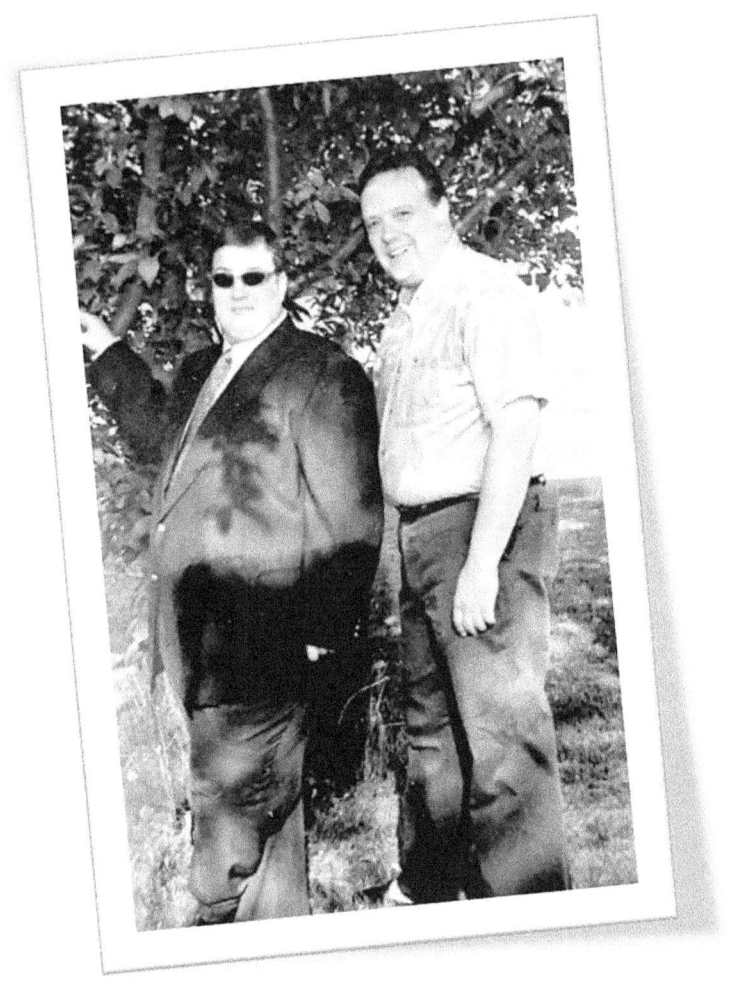

With Josh on his Graduation Day in 2002, Marla is behind the camera.

Life's Journey Extended

By age nineteen, he started to tire of fighting for a normal life. He had always had to work harder than most for everything. Just a year earlier when, a learning support advisor wanted him to take a higher-level math class as a senior. Josh pleaded with me. "Dad, I'm just tired." I understood what he meant. For years, he had spent two to three hours a night on what other students could often complete in half the time, but like a trooper, he had done it. I told his advisor, "No, he'll take the basic math class he needs." The advisor wasn't happy, but Josh just wanted to enjoy his senior year, and it certainly wasn't going to improve his educational or career possibilities to take a higher level of math. As sometimes happens to those with intellectual and developmental disabilities, being tired of the fight for normality led to suicidal ideations, followed by several suicide attempts for which he was hospitalized. What Josh needed most was structure and around-the-clock support. With an IQ of over 69 but under 80, Josh was not a candidate for an MR or IDD group home. One of these homes would have been the ideal placement for Josh, but his slightly higher IQ and the lack of understanding of what we now know as the autism spectrum left only mental health facilities as an option. Eventually, after several unsuccessful suicide attempts, Josh was committed to first Harrisburg and then Wernersville State Hospital. All but one of the next twelve years were spent in a state hospital with us, making regular visits to see him and taking him out on day trips and, when allowed, overnight and weekend passes.

It is a certainty that the state hospital was not the best placement for Josh. Mental health facilities are about giving the patient as many choices as possible, which only led to confusion and frustration for Josh. If things were very predictable and consistent, Josh was pleased. If things started to get unpredictable and inconsistent, Josh became anxious.

When he was anxious, Josh frequently became agitated. This agitation led to acting out, which led to heavier doses of Psychotropic meds, usually benzodiazepines. These benzodiazepines would relax him and his muscles, including the epiglottis, as we learned over time. So, off and on, from ages 22 to 26, Josh was hospitalized with chemical cases of pneumonia—some years, as high as nine times a year. The worst of those moments came in 2009 (at age 25) when his pulse ox reached a low of 40; he went into cardiac arrest and had to be intubated and put in a medically induced coma.

The pulmonologist who took care of him said, "Folks, you need to begin to prepare yourself for the day that we aren't able to bring him back." He made a rather fantastic recovery after that incident. We finally won the battle with the hospital over benzodiazepines, which we had been having for years. We told them countless times that the muscle relaxant seemed, from our observation when we were with him, to be affecting the function of his epiglottis. It wasn't until a Dr. that we explained his epiglottis history to at Reading Hospital wrote in his chart that he was "Allergic" to Benzodiazepines that they quit using them on him at the state hospital. His health began to improve, and by 2011, there was talk of a discharge to a group home. He seemed to be doing well emotionally and psychologically.

So, from 2011 to 2012, Josh lived in a group home in Pottsville, PA, just minutes from our house. He was able to attend church with us from time to time at Kimmel's Church in Orwigsburg, PA. We enjoyed having Josh in the community with us, but as he reached the one-year mark, the group home wanted to start looking for a transition into apartment living for him. Just discussing this elevated Josh's anxieties to the point that he became involved in self-harm.

Despite a year of success in the group home and a valiant effort to live in the community, Josh needed a more structured environment than an apartment of his own. After a series of brief hospitalizations in 2012, he was committed to the State Hospital in Danville, PA. Something he said when he was readmitted to the state hospital didn't make sense until after his passing. He said, "Dad, I just feel like this is where I belong. No, I don't always like how things go, but I need to be here." As parents who wanted so much more for their son, it was hard to hear him say that.

We went back to visiting him regularly in a state hospital and taking him out for day passes and weekends when allowed. By this point in Josh's life, he was also beginning to experience the effects of his numerous bouts of "chemical" pneumonia, which made him more susceptible to infection and upper respiratory problems. We did our best to keep an eye on his health since, at times, he was not the best at self-advocacy or reporting his health issues to the staff. While he was no longer receiving benzodiazepines, he was back to being exposed to more potential causes of infection in the group environment of a state hospital.

During this time, when he wasn't battling recurrent episodes of upper respiratory infection and pneumonia, he must have been carrying on his own hospital ministry. Occasionally, I would get a call where he would ask me to send him another Bible. Then, there were the calls where he asked fairly deep theological questions. I did my best to answer his questions and send or bring him the resources he was asking for, and we both kept in regular contact with him from 2012 to 2016. Despite the countless times we had seen his life dangle from a fragile thread, still, nothing had prepared either of us for the call Marla received from the state hospital staff on March 23, 2016. While experiencing respiratory difficulties brought on by a bout with MERS (Middle Eastern Respiratory Syndrome – COVID 2015), our son entered cardiac arrest in the lobby of the state hospital while on his way to the emergency room at Geisinger Hospital in Danville, PA. The staff was unable to revive him. Nothing prepares a parent for the loss of a child. You don't get over the loss in time. At best, you learn to live with the loss by finding meaning and purpose in the life of the child you loved and raised. Finding that meaning and purpose allows you to comfort yourself while you wait to be reunited with the child you love.

I didn't know what was going on behind this picture until we attended a memorial service that was held for him by the patients and staff at the state hospital. When we met with the hospital chaplain, we were told about Josh's ministry to other patients and staff when he wasn't struggling. It seemed that Josh had impacted as many and perhaps more lives in the state hospital system than he had impacted during the 19 years he lived in our home. It became clear to

Marla and me that the State Hospital had been yet another mission field for him.

The disciples asked Jesus,

> "Rabbi who sinned, this man or his parents, that he was born blind?"
>
> "Neither this man nor his parents sinned," said Jesus, "but this happened so the works of God might be displayed in him."

I finally have come to accept that while I, as an earthly father, would have chosen a different quality of life for my son, his Heavenly Father had other plans and used Josh to bring Glory and Honor to his Name for over 31 years.

If I had any lingering doubts about this, those doubts were washed away during our planning for his celebration of life service. As I looked over his life and the photographs and reflected on the people whose lives had been touched by Josh, I knew God's plan for our son's life had been fulfilled. During that planning, Christ showed up again and brought me back to that moment of divine appointment in the hospital examining room with Doctor Legend. While discussing a gravesite with Dr. Landon (not his name), a member of the church we were attending, I shared with him the story of Josh's experience with

Dr Legend. I didn't know then and never could have expected that Dr. Landon, a now-retired successful plastic surgeon living in Pennsylvania, had interned in surgery under Dr. Legend at the University of Minnesota over 20 years earlier. When Dr. Landon shared his experience working with Dr. Legend as his head intern just a few years after Josh's stay in Minneapolis, it sent shivers through me. It clarified that God knew who we were, where we were, and what we needed. Just as He had spoken through Dr. Legend in that hospital room over 30 years earlier and extended Josh's life and ministry, He was now helping us arrange a final resting place for our son with the assistance of a church board member who interned under Dr. Legend. The unexpected, almost unbelievable connection between these two physicians in different parts of the country and many years apart was God's subtle way of sending me the message that he still knew who we were, where we were, and what we were going through.

For more than thirty-one years the works of God were manifested in Josh's life in various ways and settings. Numerous individuals saw God's Glorious hand in our son's life. Commitments to Christ from school psychologists, bus drivers, and community members resulted from his heart for ministry. Often, he didn't know how to finish up with them, and Mom or I, in the case of the school psychologist, got called in, but he was utterly fearless when it came to sharing the love of Christ with those around him. I still remember someone years ago who wanted to be sympathetic, saying, "I don't know how you do it – raising a son with special needs. I couldn't do it. He is lucky to have the two of you."

I said, "I'm the lucky one. It has been a privilege to be Josh's father. I am a better man for having been given that privilege."

In the forty years since those men offered that prayer of faith over our son, I have prayed for healing and deliverance for countless people around the altars of numerous churches. It has been my privilege to witness God's hand working in mighty and miraculous ways. Despite a deep sense of personal loss following Josh's passing on March 23, 2016, I still believe that Jesus Christ is:

> *"the same yesterday, and today, and forever."*
> *(Hebrews 13:8)*

Anything God ever has done, He is still doing because he does not change. In short, I still believe in the power of prayer. I still believe the Prayer of Faith works.

Healing here on earth can look different from person to person and from situation to situation. Healing from the minor maladies of life may provide instant relief for the person in need. Then there are those more long-term and terminal diagnoses. The question often arises during a discussion of praying for the sick – Why does God heal one person with a long-term or terminal illness and seem to, from our perspective, ignore another person? The story of King Hezekiah illustrates something God has been telling us all along. The Prophet Isaiah writes:

> *In those days was Hezekiah sick unto death. And Isaiah the prophet the son of Amoz came unto him, and said to him, Thus saith the Lord, Set thine house in order: for thou shalt die, and not live. Isaiah 38:1 (KJV)*

Notice that the beginning of this verse says King Hezekiah was "sick unto death." The idea of being "sick unto death" is a subtle reminder of a profound Biblical truth.

> *"It is appointed unto men once to die." Hebrews 9:27 (KJV)*

We each have an appointment with death. While none of us know the day or the hour of that appointment, you can be confident you have an appointment.

For Hezekiah, his time had arrived. Isaiah told the King, perhaps one of Israel's most righteous kings up to that point, to get his affairs in order. Hezekiah, you don't have long. You are going to die. Hezekiah was terminal, as we would call it; he was "sick unto death."

Recognizing that we are all going to die should give us a different perspective on terminal illness than it frequently does. Since it is appointed unto all of us once to die, healing for the terminally ill involves life extension and not the promise of living forever in this mortal flesh. So, when Hezekiah received from Dr. Isaiah the news of his impending death

> *Then Hezekiah turned his face toward the wall, and prayed unto the Lord, and said, remember now, O Lord, I beseech thee, How I have walked before thee in truth and with a perfect heart, and have done that which is good in thy sight. And Hezekiah wept sore. Isaiah 38:2-3 (KJV)*

God reviewed his case and sent Isaiah back to Hezekiah with the following message in Isaiah 38:5 (KJV):

> *Thus, saith the Lord, the God of David thy father, I have heard thy prayer, I have seen thy tears: behold, I will add unto thy days fifteen years.*

God granted Hezekiah a fifteen-year life extension. What is evident here is that God decided to postpone Hezekiah's appointment, not Isaiah and certainly not Hezekiah.

> **Like King Hezekiah You Can:**
> **OUTLIVE EVERY PROGNOSIS THROUGH THE POWER OF PRAYER!**

We live in a world where everyone seems to want a guarantee. When it comes to healing and your health, the only absolute guarantee is that someday you will die. That someday, I have come to believe, is closely tied to your life's eternal purpose. Yes, I believe each of us has a divine purpose here on earth. Whether or not you discover and follow your God-given purpose, you still have one.

If everyone is not healed here on earth, why pray for the sick? Simply put, we still don't know, even with all our modern medical technology and advances, when this or that person is going to die. We may see that they have a sickness that usually leads to death, but like Isaiah, we don't know the exact time of their death, and we also don't know if God may, in his infinite wisdom, decide to extend their life.

At the end of the day, though, healing is not our work but the work of the Holy Spirit working in and through us. When we offer the prayer of faith over the sick, we invite the indwelling presence of God, the Holy Spirit living inside us, to rise up within us, speak through us, and touch that person at the point of their need. Please notice here that while we may be anointing the sick with oil and praying over them, God is still the One doing the work, not us.

Jesus is still telling us, like he told the father in Mark Chapter 9, that He can still do anything through us. Jesus told that father when the father asked Him if He could heal his son since the disciples couldn't, "If thou canst believe, all things are possible to him that believeth." (Mark 9:23 KJV) The New Living Translation gives some insight into this verse in the following

> *"What do you mean, 'If I Can'?" Jesus asked. "Anything is possible if a person believes." Mark 9:23 (NLT)*

The unspoken but intended last three words of that last sentence are "with God's help." Jesus challenges the man's uncertainty about whether or not He could or would heal his son. We, like that man, need to cry out for our sons and

LIFE'S JOURNEY EXTENDED

our daughters, our friends, our neighbors, and those who ask for us to pray with them like that father so long ago:

> ***I do believe; help me*** *overcome my unbelief!*
> *Mark 9:24 (NIV)*

All Done!

In the fall of 1979, I stood looking over the ruins of what was once ancient Jericho, listening to our guide describe the grandeur of a walled fortress city so large that the walls themselves were wide enough to carry two chariots side by side. Jericho was undoubtedly the most entrenched fortress city the early Israeli warriors faced. Its walls were daunting. The battles we face in the spiritual world as couples are often no less daunting. To us, they are a real challenge to our faith.

As I looked at what was left of the ancient city of Jericho, I was reminded of how God spoke to Joshua, the General, and leader of the nation of Israel and its army. The Biblical account is found in Joshua Chapter 6:

> *And the Lord said unto Joshua, See, I have given into thine hand Jericho, and the king thereof, and the mighty men of valour. And ye shall compass the city, all ye men of war, and go round about the city once. Thus shalt thou do six*

> *days. And seven priests shall bear before the ark seven trumpets of rams' horns: and the seventh day ye shall compass the city seven times, and the priests shall blow with the trumpets. And it shall come to pass, that when they make a long blast with the ram's horn, and when ye hear the sound of the trumpet, all the people shall shout with a great shout; and the wall of the city shall fall down flat, and the people shall ascend up every man straight before him... Joshua 6:2-5 (KJV)*

The final verse in this story tells us that when the people followed God's plan:

> *the wall fell down flat, so that the people went up into the city, every man straight before him, and they took the city. Joshua 6:20 (KJV)*

As our guide explained how those massive walls fell or were swallowed up by the ground, she told us that the collapse of the walls was doubtless an example of the effects of sonics on that massive structure. Our guide reminded us of a famous 1970s television commercial for Memorex® Audio Cassettes. In that commercial singer, Ella Fitzgerald's voice was used to demonstrate the power of sonics. To demonstrate the reliability of their tape, Memorex® showed you Ms. Fitzgerald hitting a high note both live and on tape and shattering a wine glass both ways, and asked, "Is it live, or is it Memorex®?" Either way, live or recorded, the fall of the walls of Jericho and the gracious life extension God gave our son are examples of miracles that need to be remembered.

Yes, sonics doubtless played a part in the fall of the walls of Jericho. That does not make their fall less miraculous when you consider Joshua had no scientists in his camp and had no way of knowing how this would all work. All he had was a word from the Lord and a simple childlike belief that if God says it, He will do it.

Remember, Joshua and Caleb, whom Moses sent out to spy on the land 40 years earlier, were the only two out of 12 spies who believed God would give them the Promised Land. While the other ten spies shrunk in fear, Joshua and Caleb offered a "good report" that the land was flowing with "milk and honey" and could be taken by Israel. As a result of Israel's UNBELIEF, they wandered in the desert for forty years until the entire generation of those spies died off, except for Joshua and Caleb. We named our son Joshua because, in my mind, the biblical Joshua and Caleb were the kind of men I wanted my sons to become. While Marla would not

ALL DONE!

agree to naming our younger son Caleb when he was born in 1986, Jacob possesses the same optimism and tenacity as Caleb. Like his older brother, Jacob reminds me daily, through his creativity and hard work, how proud and thankful I am to have had the privilege of being their father.

In one of his final journal entries, before he passed in 2016, Joshua profoundly drove home just how much he understood the responsibility to accept God at His Word and "soldier on," even when the path seemed unclear and the future uncertain. Speaking of David and his battle as a youth with Goliath, Josh wrote:

> *"I can't imagine what would have happened if David would have stopped and took a minute to think about what he was going to do. He could have DIED! When God prompts us to do something, we need to respond right away!"*
>
> Joshua David Langley

OUTLIVE EVERY PROGNOSIS

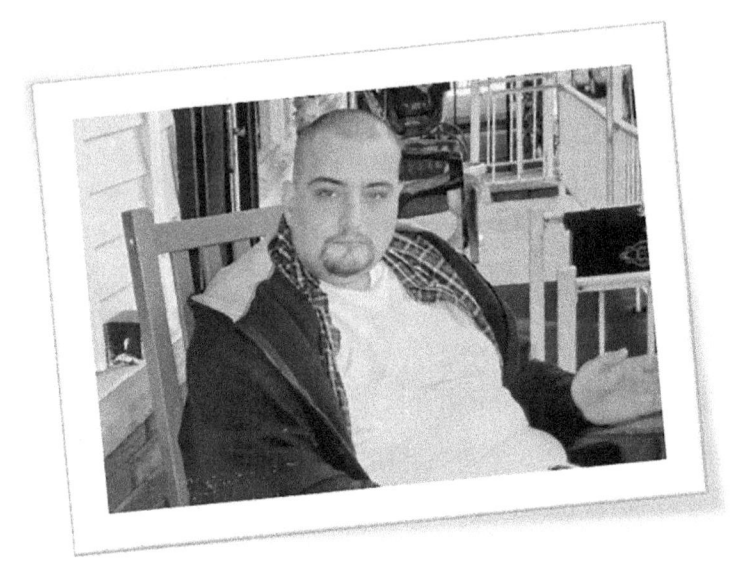

The goodbye wave in our last good picture of Josh, probably taken in 2012, hangs on our office wall as a reminder of just how much he is missed!

No matter what a medical professional has told you or someone you love, please let me assure you that Jesus Christ is "the same yesterday, and to day, and for ever."

> **You or They can:
> OUTLIVE EVERY PROGNOSIS THROUGH
> THE POWER OF PRAYER!**

Author's Afterword

My journey has taught me that while many of us can tell stories of our own less-than-ideal beginnings, life is not about how we start but how we finish. Rooted in the sincere conviction that every life has a God-given purpose, I believe how we respond to that purpose ("our calling") is abundantly important. The recognition and pursuit of our God-given purpose should lead us to strive and reach for "the prize of the high calling of God in Christ Jesus." (Philippians 3:14 KJV) That "prize" of which Paul speaks is, I believe, hearing the words at the climax of our journey:

> *"Well done, thou good and faithful servant: thou hast been faithful over a few things, I will make thee ruler over many things: enter thou into the joy of thy Lord" Matthew 25:21 KJV*

For Josh, the journey included both physical and mental health challenges. I tried here to share his physical health story to explain what his journey taught us all about the healing and life extension available through the shed blood of Jesus Christ. I could not begin here to describe the lessons we learned about defeating the darkness and navigating the mental health system as parents and believers. I have left that and some of our grieving for my next book.

From Author:

DAVE LANGLEY

Coming in November of 2025:

DEFEAT
THE DARKNESS

"If you or someone you love struggle with depression, experience separation anxiety, social anxiety, suicidal ideation, have an active mental health diagnosis, have spent time in a mental health facility, or battle dark emotional, psychological, or spiritual forces, this book is for you!"